The Simple Six

THE EASY WAY TO GET IN SHAPE AND STAY IN
SHAPE FOR THE REST OF YOUR LIFE

CLINTON DOBBINS

DISCLAIMER

You should consult your physician or other health care professional before starting this or any other fitness program to determine if it is right for your needs. This is particularly true if you (or your family) have a history of high blood pressure or heart disease, or if you have ever experienced chest pain when exercising or have experienced chest pain in the past month when not engaged in physical activity, smoke, have high cholesterol, are obese, or have a bone or joint problem that could be made worse by a change in physical activity. Do not start this fitness program if your physician or health care provider advises against it. If you experience faintness, dizziness, pain or shortness of breath at any time while exercising you should stop immediately.

CONTENTS

THE SIMPLE SIX

1

INTRODUCTION

No pain, no gain has been a rallying cry in the fitness world for decades.

I get it, intense workouts are seductive. It's easy to get caught up in the energy and hype of high intensity training (HIT) or high volume weight lifting sessions. Adding 5 more pounds, pushing out one more rep, giving it your all and collapsing in a pool of sweat. It's a romantic idea and finishing a hard workout can provide a great sense of accomplishment.

But intense exercise takes a lot out of you. Any one session can leave you feeling drained and tired for the rest of the day, and residual soreness can keep you from wanting to work out again the next day or even the next week.

Frequent intense exercise sessions can lead to exhaustion, expose you to a higher risk of injury due to overuse and increased impact to the muscles and joints, and may ultimately result in failure.

High intensity, high volume workout programs also come with a caveat that is rarely mentioned in the brochure. Most people start an exercise program expecting to lose a few pounds. And it's easy to think that if you work out harder you'll lose weight faster. The truth is that if you want to succeed at a high intensity, high volume training program, then you must fuel up for a high intensity, high volume training program. Your diet must be structured in a way that supports the demands you're asking of your body. This means increasing calories, especially carbohydrates, to match the energy output required to get through your training. This is all well and good if training is your first priority, but if you also intend to diet or follow any type of restricted eating plan then be very careful not to overexert your system by trying to do too much.

I don't mean to take anything away from those who enjoy HIT style workouts. There should be room for everyone at the table when it comes to fitness and helping people lead healthier lifestyles. I have close friends who are involved with Crossfit and have seen firsthand the positive impact they've had on the lives of the many wonderful people in their communities. I was a member of a Crossfit gym myself for a couple of years and enjoyed the environment and the challenge it provided. However, as time went on I found that the considerable demands on my time and on my body meant that it just wasn't a sustainable program for me.

If we're being honest with ourselves, then I'm willing to bet that high intensity or high volume workout programs aren't sustainable for most people. The demands on your body and your time are simply too high. These workouts are designed to take a lot out of you; unfortunately they often take too much.

When programed and performed correctly an exercise program should give you more energy and ability than it takes away! That's the real secret to creating an exercise program that is sustainable for years to come, and it's what I set out to accomplish with The Simple Six.

The Simple Six is an innovative new workout program designed to provide maximum results with the least amount of effort.

The unique programming method found only in The Simple Six is based on the idea that repeating a small amount of work consistently can lead to great changes in the way you look, the way you feel, and the way you think about fitness and exercise.

If you're looking for a simple, straightforward way to build a strong, balanced, and capable physique, then The Simple Six is for you.

The Simple Six truly is the easy way to get in shape and stay in shape for the rest of your life!

Enjoy!

2

THE SIMPLE SIX

The guiding principle behind The Simple Six program is that consistency outperforms intensity.

This program was created with the long game in mind. By consistently putting in small amounts of work, over time you will see the same (or better) results as from any high intensity program. Best of all, these results aren't temporary; this program is meant to last a lifetime.

So what is The Simple Six?

The Simple Six is a minimalist exercise program designed to:

- Be a viable, long term exercise program for anyone regardless of age or ability

- Provide a full body workout that will increase strength and improve cardiovascular health

- Improve body composition by adding muscle and reducing fat

- Produce the best possible results with the least amount of effort

Too many workout programs focus on specific muscles or exercises. "The Top 5 Moves for Bigger Biceps!", "Add 50 Pounds to Your Deadlift This Month!" Yeah okay, whatever you say supplement company sponsored bodybuilding magazine.

The Simple Six focuses on a minimal set of basic exercises, and each of these exercises focuses on one of the basic human movement patterns. These are natural movements or motions that the human body is built to perform. Train each movement pattern, and you will be rewarded with a strong, balanced, and capable physique.

The six exercises included in The Simple Six program target the following movement patterns:

- Squat

- Hinge

- Push (Horizontal)

- Push (Vertical)

- Pull

- Gait

Wait a minute... You're telling me the entire program is only six exercises?!?!

Yep, that's what I'm telling you. The entire point of The Simple Six is to offer a simple and straight forward program that can provide sustainable results and continue helping build a healthier and more capable you for years to come. That means sticking to basic, proven exercises and programming them in a way that maximizes their benefit.

"Perfection is achieved, not when there is nothing more to add,
but when there is nothing left to take away."

- Antoine de Saint-Exupéry

Remember, more isn't always better. In the same way that consistency can outperform intensity; simplicity can outperform complexity.

3

A WORD ON CONSISTENCY

"More" is a very popular word in the health and fitness industry.

Personal trainers and online gurus are falling all over themselves promising to turn you into more than you are today. They guarantee more muscle, more fat loss, more sex appeal; but only if you're willing to give more time, more effort, more blood, sweat and tears (and more money!).

"More isn't always better, Linus. Sometimes it's just more."

\- Sabrina (1995)

The truth is that for most people who are trying to get into or stay in shape there is only one "more" that will allow them to reach their goals... More consistency!

Consistency is the difference between failure and success in almost every aspect of life, but especially so when it comes to your health.

It isn't enough to diet for 30 days or to complete a 6 week training program. If you want to live a long, healthy life then you need to adopt a long-term, healthy lifestyle.

Part of that lifestyle should be daily exercise. This exercise doesn't have to be too hard or take too long, it just has to become a part of your routine. There will be days when you'll feel good and be excited to exercise, and there will be days when exercise is the last thing on your mind. The important thing is to be sure you do a little bit each day. Over time these days turn into weeks, then into months and years.

I understand that life sometimes gets in the way. You're sick, have family commitments, get caught up at work. It happens. Try to develop an 80/20 mindset. If you make the right choices and follow your routine 80% of the time, then the remaining 20% won't hurt your results in the long run. So if you miss a day or even a few days don't sweat it, just get back as soon as possible and pick up right where you left off.

Imagine if you were to follow an exercise program to the letter for the next month. How much better would you look and feel? What if you did that program for the next year? The next 2 years? The next 10?

That's what I'm offering with The Simple Six. A small amount of work, repeated consistently, that can lead to great changes in the way you look and feel... Forever!

And it all starts today!

4

THE SQUAT

Squatting might be the most fundamental movement pattern we have in our human repertoire. Squatting is such an instinctual and natural position for humans. It is one of our first movements and we are able to execute a perfect squat right out of the gate. Babies are the world's greatest squatters. I get jealous watching a baby squat. They can get their butts all the way to the ground so effortlessly and comfortably.

Squatting is literally something we were born to do.

Unfortunately in today's world squatting isn't something we continue to do throughout our lives. At a young age we trade in squatting for sitting. Sitting in chairs, sitting at desks, sitting in cars, sitting on couches. The older we get, the more we sit.

Without repetition, our bodies quickly forget that we are supposed to be able to squat effortlessly. Our hips, knees, and ankles tighten, the muscles in our legs weaken and shorten, and we lose the flexibility and balance required to drop our butts to the ground without falling over.

But hope is not lost. We can all still squat; we just have to remember how. Fortunately, it's easy. The secret to remembering how to squat well is, well, to squat.

When most people think about the squat as an exercise, they probably think about the barbell back squat. While that is certainly the most famous variation of the squat, it isn't the only one and (Spoiler Alert) it isn't the variation I recommend.

For one thing, the barbell back squat requires a barbell. You'll also need a squat rack to hold that bar, a large amount of plates to load weight onto it, and a space to fit it all in. Not to mention, a fair amount of strength and

7

technique in order to perform the exercise safely and effectively.

The Simple Six is a minimalist program. That means the exercises included in the program should be readily available to most people in most places. It's important that these exercises are not only extremely effective, but also require relatively minimal amounts of equipment, expertise, time, and money.

So I'm not recommending that you jump under a loaded barbell and start back squatting. I'm recommending that you simply start doing what you were born to do, bend at the knees and lower yourself down into the squatting position.

Which brings us to the first exercise in The Simple Six...

5

THE GOBLET SQUAT

The goblet squat is one of the simplest and most effective exercises you can do. The goblet squat is a full body exercise. It strengthens your quads, calves and glutes, works your core, and even helps improve your arm and grip strength because you're holding the weight in your hands.

Unlike heavier squat variations in which form or range of motion can be compromised in order to stabilize a loaded barbell, the goblet squat can actually help to improve and reinforce the movement pattern of the squat.

By holding a relatively light weight at your chest you are providing a counterbalance that will help reinforce proper posture and alignment during the squat. Because of this counterbalance, the goblet squat has a much shorter learning curve than other squat variations, allowing people of all ages and abilities to safely perform the exercise properly.

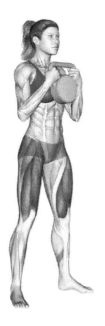
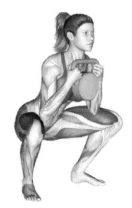

To perform the goblet squat:

1. Start by holding a relatively light dumbbell, kettlebell, or plate at your chest with both hands. Your feet should be about shoulder width apart.

2. Brace your core and begin the movement by reaching your butt back and down, as if you were about to sit in a chair. While keeping your chest up and your back straight, continue lowering yourself down as far as you can. Over time, work to get lower and lower in the bottom position, slowly increasing hip mobility until you're able to go into a full, deep squat.

3. From the bottom of the squat, drive from your heels and rise back to standing. Make sure that your knees, butt, and back are all moving at the same speed so that you maintain an upright posture throughout the entire movement.

Side Note

Everyone's foot placement is unique, and a little shift in positon can make a big difference. To find your optimal foot placement, perform three vertical jumps as quickly as you can and note where your feet land after the third jump. This is your natural positioning and you should mimic this foot placement during your squats.

Just starting out?

Try one of these squatting exercises, perfect for beginners or those with physical limitations that might impair this movement pattern:

- Shallow Knee Bends

- Chair or Box Squats

- Bodyweight Squats to Parallel

- Deep Bodyweight Squats

6

THE HINGE

The hinge, or hip hinge, is one of the most important movement patterns for overall health and wellbeing. Sadly, it's also one of the most neglected. Humans today spend an unfortunate amount of time sitting. The seated position puts a lot of strain on the back muscles and the spine. It also leads to tight hamstrings and hip flexors. All of this can wreck your posture and contribute heavily to low back pain. There are over 3 million medical cases of low back pain reported in the US each year, and undoubtedly millions of more people worldwide who suffer from low back pain every day.

Luckily, low back pain associated with sitting all day is a self-treatable condition, and the best treatment option is to practice exercises that incorporate the hinge.

Hinge exercises are particularly useful given our modern, chair-based lifestyle. Properly training the hinge will strengthen the entire posterior chain, the group of muscles along the back of your body that includes the hamstrings and glutes as well as the muscles of the mid and low back. Hinge exercises also teach and reinforce proper hip extension, which goes a long way in correcting many of the postural and low back issues that plague society.

The most famous of the hinge exercises is the deadlift. Simply put, a deadlift is when you reach down to grab a loaded barbell and then stand up straight to lift the weight from the ground to about waist high. The deadlift is a tremendous full body exercise. It works all the major muscle groups and engages more muscles than any other exercise (including the squat!). There's an argument to be made that if you could only do one exercise for the rest of your life then it should be the deadlift.

So I'm recommending the deadlift as the Simple Six hinge exercise right? Wrong. Much like the barbell squat, the deadlift requires more equipment and expertise than is necessary. Why do with more what can be done with less?

Why do with more what can be done with a kettlebell...

7

THE KETTLEBELL SWING

A Kettlebell is a beautiful thing!

For those of you who are unfamiliar, a kettlebell is a cast-iron ball with a handle attached. Basically, it's a cannonball with a handle. Kettlebells have been used in Russia by strongmen for hundreds of years.

Kettlebells can be used in a variety of ways, but they really stand out when used for ballistic exercise. Ballistic exercises are exercises that combine strength, cardio, and flexibility training in a single, dynamic movement. When it comes to getting the most bang for your buck, it's hard to beat ballistic exercises. And when it comes to ballistic exercises, it's hard to beat the kettlebell swing.

The kettlebell swing isn't just a full body exercise. It's what I like to call a full body response exercise. With this single exercise you will:

- Strengthen the muscles of the posterior trail

- Develop stronger and more symmetrical core muscles

- Build stronger, wider lats and shoulders

- Increase strength in your grip, wrists, and forearms

- Develop power and explosiveness in your hips

- Supercharge muscle endurance and aerobic capacity

- Reduce low back pain and protect your low back from injury

- Burn serious amounts of body fat

It's safe to say that I'm a big fan of the kettlebell swing. In fact, if I could only do one exercise for the rest of my life, I would choose the kettlebell swing without hesitation.

For The Simple Six we're focusing on the two handed kettlebell swing.

Side Note

The single arm kettlebell swing is a great exercise as well. It provides all the same benefits of the two handed swing, but adds an anti-rotational component that really amps up core stabilization. Once you master the two handed swing, feel free to experiment with single arm swings if you'd like.

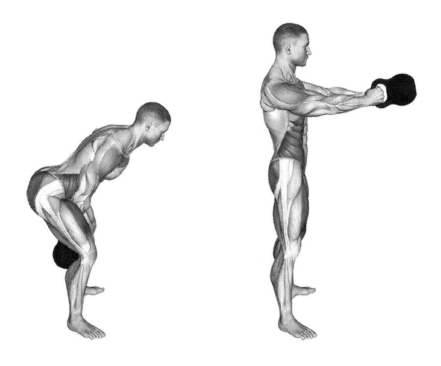

To perform the two handed kettlebell swing:

1. Place your feet slightly wider than shoulder width and point your toes out just a bit. Your weight should remain in the middle of the feet and your knees should track in line with your toes throughout the movement.

2. Setup the kettlebell about a foot in front of your toes.

3. Comfortably grip the bell with both hands. You should hold the bell so that it's only slightly loose in your hands. Too tight of a grip can cause blisters and too loose of a grip could cause the bell to slip out of your hands.

4. To start the swing, hike the kettlebell back between your legs so that your forearms meet your inner thigh and the bell is extended behind your butt.

5. Use your hips to drive the kettlebell back through your legs and

up until your arms extend horizontally out in front of you.

6. As the kettlebell falls, control it back through your legs to the starting position.

A few helpful tips for the kettlebell swing.

- Remember that the swing is a hinge movement, not a squat, so the shins should stay mostly vertical. Instead of bending at the knees you should be reaching your butt back as you lower to the kettlebell.

- It's important to brace your core and keep your back straight throughout the entire movement. Make sure you really work to tighten your abs in order to keep your mid-section in a straight line.

- The hips should be moving the kettlebell, not the arms or shoulders. Your arms should be acting only to hold the bell, not to raise it. Keep your shoulders in a relaxed but stable position and the kettlebell swing will reward you with increased shoulder flexibility and range of motion.

- Once you finish a set a swings, always let the kettlebell come to a complete rest before setting it back down on the ground. The last thing you want is for a kettlebell to go flying across the room.

- Make sure that the area around you is clear before you start swinging. Kettlebells are hard and heavy; you don't want kids or pets coming into the path of the kettlebell unexpectedly!

Side Note

The kettlebell swing is a simple concept, but the execution of a good swing is fairly complex. If you're new to kettlebells (or could use a refresher) I highly recommend heading over to YouTube to watch a few videos on proper kettlebell swing form and mechanics.

Just starting out?

Try one of these hinge exercises, perfect for beginners or those with physical limitations that might impair this movement pattern:

- Bodyweight Good Mornings

- Hip Raise or Basic Bridge

- Kettlebell Deadlift

8

THE PUSH

If you've ever been a member of a commercial gym, you know that Monday is national bench press day. The bench press has become so ubiquitous that when you ask someone how much they lift, they will immediately respond with their max bench press weight.

Needless to say, the push movement has been over prioritized in the fitness world for decades. So much so, that many people neglect other movement patterns like the pull or hinge in order to pursue a heavier and heavier bench press. So how does The Simple Six help to combat this lack of balance and over emphasis on the push? By making it the only movement pattern we recommend two exercises for of course!

Okay, so if the push has been overdone to the detriment of other movements then why am I recommending two exercises for the push? Because there are two distinct planes in which the push can operate.

Horizontal pushes, like the bench press, involve pushing a weight out in front of your body.

Vertical pushing involves keeping the weight in line with your torso and pushing it straight up overhead.

While obviously similar, horizontal and vertical pushing exercises have surprisingly little overlap. They emphasize different muscles and ranges of motion, so strength in the horizontal push doesn't necessarily translate to strength in the vertical push (and vice versa).

Both horizontal and vertical pushing exercises contribute to overall upper body strength and play important roles in developing major muscle groups like the chest, shoulders, and arms. No workout program is complete without both.

9

THE PUSH-UP

The basics are the basics for a reason, they provide everything you need and don't waste your time with extra junk. Does an exercise get more basic than the push-up? I have a better question...

Does an exercise get more perfect than the push-up?

Meager as it might be considered by some, the push-up really is the quintessential minimalist exercise. The push-up is easy to learn, simple to perform, and requires no equipment whatsoever. At a moment's notice the push-up is ready to provide a workout that targets muscles in the chest, arms, and shoulders, engages your core and works your abs, and helps build stabilizer muscles throughout your entire body.

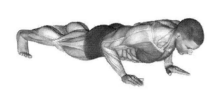 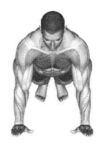

To perform a push-up:

1. Start in a plank position. Your hands should be directly under shoulders. Spread your fingers and rotate your hands out just slightly so that the "V's" created by your thumbs and first fingers are pointing forward (this helps align your arms and shoulders properly, preventing your elbows from flaring out as you lower your body). Tighten your abs, squeeze your butt, and flatten your back so your body is neutral and straight.

2. Lower your body until your chest touches the floor. Make sure you stay tight and keep a flat back. Your butt shouldn't sag or stick up; your body should stay in a straight line. Focus your eyes on a spot a foot or two in front of you to help maintain a neutral neck. Keep your elbows tucked in close and parallel to your body, don't "T" them out.

3. Push back to the starting position. Remember to keep everything engaged and tight, always maintain that straight line.

Just starting out?

Try one of these horizontal pushing exercises, perfect for beginners or those with physical limitations that might impair this movement pattern:

- Wall Push-up

- Knee Push-up

- Negative Push-up

10

THE KETTLEBELL PRESS

We've covered horizontal pushing with the push-up, so let's move on to vertical pushing.

Vertical pushing is simply pressing a weight in a straight line up and overhead. Exercises targeting this movement pattern are commonly referred to as presses, overhead presses, or shoulder presses and can make use of barbells, dumbbells, or kettlebells.

My recommendation for The Simple Six is the single arm kettlebell press.

Due the design of a kettlebell, hand positioning and the resting position for the kettlebell press differs from the barbell or dumbbell press. This is a good thing, as it lends the kettlebell press to a more natural plane of movement.

Instead of forcing you to lean out of the way of a barbell or to flare your elbows in order to accommodate a dumbbell, the kettlebell helps keep your body aligned and your elbows tight. It also forces your hand (and the weight) to the front of your body in the starting position which, in turn, creates a greater stabilization response than other press variations.

Side Note

If you've been paying attention to this point you'll notice that I've recommended kettlebell exercises a couple of times. Besides being extremely effective, kettlebells are versatile, portable, and affordable. Relying on kettlebells allows The Simple Six to stay minimal while still providing you the best results possible.

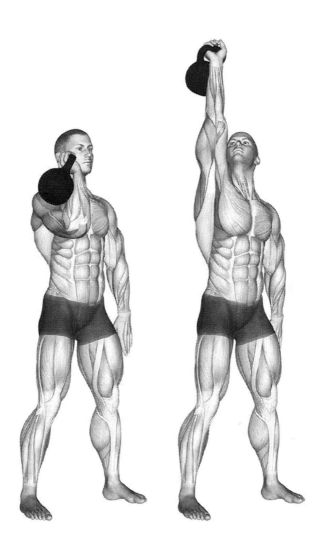

To perform the kettlebell press:

1. Clean the kettlebell to the starting position by extending your legs and hips as you pull the kettlebell up from the ground and towards your shoulder. As you raise the bell, rotate your wrist so your palm faces inward. Your wrist should be strong and

straight, not bent, and the kettlebell should rest comfortably in the crook of your elbow around chest high.

2. Stabilize your body by squeezing your butt and bracing your core.

3. Look at the kettlebell and press it up and overhead. Make sure to keep your wrist locked in a straight line.

4. Slowly lower the kettlebell back down under control and repeat.

Just starting out?

Try one of these vertical pushing exercises, perfect for beginners or those with physical limitations that might impair this movement pattern:

- Door Stretch
- Ultra-light Shoulder Press (1-5 pound weight)
- Wall Press-up

11

THE PULL

Just like the push, the pull can be done both horizontally and vertically. Horizontal pulling exercises, like rows, are done by pulling a weight toward your body perpendicularly. Vertical pulls, like lat pull downs, involve pulling a weight down from overhead in line with your body.

Also, just like the push, both horizontal and vertical pushing exercises contribute to overall upper body strength and play important roles in developing major muscle groups; only this time we're talking about the back, shoulders, biceps and forearms.

Unlike the push however, I only recommend a single exercise for the pull movement pattern. Why is that?

First, we are already indirectly working the major muscle groups of the back with the kettlebell swing and the kettlebell press.

Second, and more importantly, there is an exercise that allows us to develop every pulling muscle with a single movement...

12

THE CHIN-UP

The chin-up is a foundational upper body strength exercise. There is a reason that chin-ups are used as a measure of basic physical fitness by numerous organizations around the world. Chin-ups are as simple of an exercise as you can find, but they aren't easy.

In order to complete even a single chin-up, you'll need a good amount of strength relative to your bodyweight. When added to a well-rounded exercise routine like The Simple Six, chin-ups will provide all the upper body muscle and strength you will ever need.

Why chin-ups instead of pull-ups, and what's the difference?

The chin-up and the pull-up are very similar. The only mechanical difference between the two is the grip. During a chin-up, you grip the bar with your palms facing toward you. For a pull-up you grip the bar with your palms facing away from you.

The reason I recommend the chin-up is that turning your palms toward you brings the biceps more into play. In fact, in my opinion, the chin-up is the best exercise you can do to build bigger, stronger biceps. Pull-ups are great too, as they put more emphasis on contraction of the mid-back. But since we're already indirectly working the back during other exercises in The Simple Six, I'll happily trade extra activation of the back muscles for extra strength and muscle growth in the biceps.

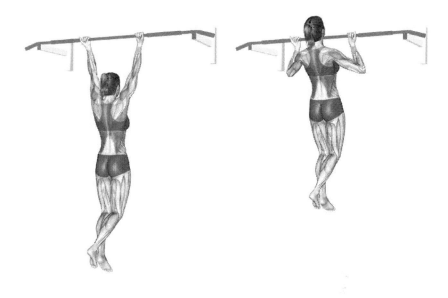

To perform the chin-up:

1. Grab the pullup bar with your hands about shoulder width apart and your palms toward you.

2. Hang from the bar with your arms fully extended.

3. Pull yourself up by squeezing your lats hard and pulling your elbows down toward the floor.

4. Raise yourself all the way up until your chin passes the bar.

5. Slowly lower yourself down until your arms are straight.

Just starting out?

Try one of these pulling exercises, perfect for beginners or those with physical limitations that might impair this movement pattern:

- Bent Over Row

- Bodyweight Row (Aussie Pull-up)

- Negative Pull-up

13

THE GAIT

Gait is nothing more than a fancy word for the movement we use to walk.

Walking isn't just a human movement pattern. Walking is THE human movement pattern. It is literally how we get from point A to point B. It's how we as a species were able to spread to and inhabit every continent on Earth (sorry Earth). Millions of years before we were bench pressing, crossfitting, or zumba-ing, we were walking.

Over the course a lifetime, we humans spend more time walking than practicing every other movement pattern combined.

So why is walking ignored in almost every exercise program ever created? Simple, it's too simple!

Walking is embraced for relaxation, rehabilitation, and as a starting point for people struggling with obesity or physical impairment. But walking as a performance exercise that burns fat and builds aerobic capacity...not a chance.

Well I'm a firm believer that walking is a performance building, fat burning rock star of an exercise, and I'll go door to door if necessary to convince the world that I'm right.

The beautiful thing about walking is that you'll feel better after you finish a walk, not worse. That isn't something you can say about high intensity cardio training. If an exercise not only gives you terrific results but leaves you full of energy and wanting to do it again the next day, then that's an exercise that you simply can't afford to leave out of your routine.

If you're willing to put fitness dogma and your own ego to the side and embrace walking as the foundation of your workout program, then I promise you this - You will look and feel better (and younger) than you ever thought possible, and that will stay with you for the rest of your life. If you keep it up!

"The journey of a thousand miles begins with one step."

- Lao Tzu

14

WALKING

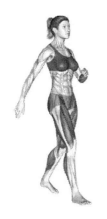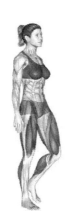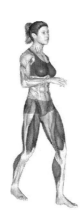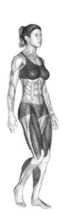

To perform the walk:

1. Put one foot in front of the other.

2. Repeat.

End of chapter.

Okay, not so fast... Walking as it fits into The Simple Six isn't quite as straight forward as opening the front door and heading out to drag your Yorkie around the neighborhood.

For The Simple Six, I'm going to give you three options when it comes to walking. Which you choose is up to you. It really depends on what your goals are, what your current ability level is, and how you feel on any given day.

Which option you choose is less important than getting up and moving a little bit every day. In the long run all that movement will add up. You'll have more energy and less stress, which will lead to a happier, healthier you!

OPTION 1 - NICE & EASY

Remember that Yorkie that needs a good dragging around? Well here's your chance. The first option for walking is just to take a casual stroll. Walk around the block, around the park, around the office, wherever you happen to be. Walk as far as you'd like and as fast (or slow) as you'd like. Just walk.

Walking consistently couldn't be simpler, couldn't be easier, and couldn't make you feel better. It will help work out any physical kinks and imbalances you're dealing with, but the biggest benefit of walking might not be physical at all.

Mental health, depression, anxiety, stress. Whatever you want to call it. We all have a ton of pressure building up inside of our heads. Walking acts as a pressure release valve for the brain and allows your thoughts and feelings to reset. You'll find that walking gives your mind a chance to work out problems or emotions you haven't been able to tie down during your day to day activities. It's also a chance to allow your creative side to thrive. Personally, some of my best ideas and breakthroughs have come during long, slow walks and I'm willing to bet the same will be true for you.

So get out there, start wandering, and see where it takes you!

OPTION 2 - UPHILL BATTLE

Walking uphill has all the benefits of regular walking, but it ratchets up your breathing, burns more fat, and increases muscle activation. It's an amazing way to raise your heart rate and build aerobic capacity without requiring the same speed, stress, and impact of other forms of cardiovascular exercise.

One of my favorite additional benefits of walking at an incline is how it helps to stretch the calves and ankles. As someone who has suffered multiple ankle injuries and fought chronic tightness in his calf muscles for longer than I can remember, I can attest to incline walking as one of the single best things you can do to help rehab and strengthen the lower legs and feet.

There are two main ways to incorporate uphill walking into your workouts. The first is pretty self-explanatory, you find a hill and you walk up it.

I'm lucky (?) to live in a rather hilly area. Near my house is a 1-mile loop that covers a relatively steep hillside. A casual walk around this loop is significantly more difficult than a flat walk, and can elicit a cardio response from even the fittest folks I know.

If you're the outdoorsy type, then head for the hills. Hiking a trail with substantial elevation changes is the perfect choice for incorporating incline training into your routine. As an extra benefit you'll get to enjoy nature and free your mind from distrac... Squirrel!!

The second option is to make use of the incline setting on a treadmill.

Didn't know your treadmill has an incline setting? You're not alone. Most people hop on a treadmill, set the speed to somewhere between jog and holy crap, then run until they hate the treadmill so much that they never go back to the gym again.

I have to stand up for the treadmill here. Sure treadmills are boring, and stupid, and boring. But besides allowing you to train comfortably at any time and in any weather, treadmills allow for a level of safety and control that you just can't get anywhere else.

Tailoring the treadmill to be the perfect companion for The Simple Six is, you guessed it, simple. Just raise the incline and start walking. For the best results find an incline setting between 5 and 10 percent that is comfortable for you, and select a speed slow enough that you can still easily carry out a conversation but fast enough that you are breathing a bit heavier than normal. For example, I prefer an 8 or 9 percent incline and a speed of 2.5 mph.

Side Note

No hill. No treadmill. No problem. Just take the stairs. Walking up and down the stairs in your home, office, or some other public place is a great substitute for incline walking!

OPTION 3 - RUCK YEAH!

Rucking is a fancy word for walking with a weighted pack on your back. It comes from the word rucksack, which is military jargon for "backpack". In the military, rucking is the foundation of physical training. Not because members of the military love rucking (trust me, they don't!), but because it's an absolute necessity that also happens to turn skinny 18 year old kids into soldiers. Elite soldiers can be responsible for carrying packs of 100 pounds or more many miles each day. Think that wouldn't lead to increased muscle endurance and fat loss??

Don't worry, I'm not trying to recruit anyone or turn you into a wannabe Special Forces operator. My goal is to offer a highly effective training method that is so simple that it's almost laughable.

Maybe some of you have been thinking "The Simple Six sounds like a great, basic workout program for some folks, but I'm looking for more than that." Well here's your chance to do more.

I know early on I said that more isn't always better. It's still true. More isn't always better, but that doesn't mean it can't be.

When you add rucking to your routine you're investing a little more effort and impact, but the return on that investment is huge.

Benefits of rucking include:

- Increased fat burning (rucking can burn 3 times more calories than walking!)

- Stronger legs, shoulders and back

- Increased endurance and heart health

- Improved posture

To get started rucking just grab a backpack. It doesn't have to be anything fancy, just pull your old Jansport out of the closet or borrow your kid's backpack and put some weight in it. Books, bricks, cans of corn, whatever. Just load it up to somewhere around 10 pounds and head out the door.

As you get used to walking with a backpack, slowly start increasing the weight. You should try to find a weight that is slightly challenging without being uncomfortable. Most people will settle into a sweet spot somewhere around 10 -15% of their bodyweight. The maximum I recommend is about 20% of your bodyweight. Anything heavier will start putting too much stress on your knees and back, and could lead to soreness or even injury in the long term. Never forget that exercise should give you more than it takes away!

Side Note

If you find that rucking is something you want to start taking seriously then have a look at backpacks and weights specifically made for rucking. They're expense but will be comfortable during even the longest rucks, which will make the activity way more enjoyable.

15

THE PROGRAM

I hope that up to this point The Simple Six has been informative and entertaining. I'm also willing to bet that I've already given you some perspective, insights, or ideas that you'll be able to take away and make a part of your training for years to come. But I'm really grateful you've stuck with me, because this is the part that I'm so excited to share with everyone.

This is where the magic happens!

Exercises don't become a workout unless they're arranged into a program, and a workout program doesn't become "The easy way to get in shape and stay in shape for the rest of your life" unless that program is innovative, easy to follow, and effective.

For The Simple Six I've done just that. By taking exercises that are highly effective on their own and combining them into a program that maximizes that effectiveness while minimizing the effort required, we're left with something truly special.

The secret that makes The Simple Six superior to other daily workout programs is a programming technique that I call ***rolling focus***.

Each day you will perform a circuit consisting of the five strength exercises covered in this book:

- The Goblet Squat
- The Kettlebell Swing
- The Push-up
- The Kettlebell Press

- The Chin-up

This circuit will be the same every day, except that each day the focus will roll on to a different one of the five exercises. Designated as **(RF)** in the plan that follows, this focus exercise will be given extra attention and will be the exercise you really want to put your energy into that day.

Every workout will give you a chance to practice the first four exercises. Use these practice sets to improve and ingrain your form and technique. You should be mostly concerned with doing these exercises correctly so as to build the muscle memory and pathways required for long term health in the associated movement patterns. Then, you will train a single exercise each day. This is your chance to sufficiently work each exercise and movement pattern weekly, allowing your body to adapt and improve in order to progress.

This rolling focus is what transforms a single daily circuit into a true full-body workout program that can provide results day after day, month after month, and year after year.

16

PROGRESSION

Progression is important for…progressing. Progression means simply adding more work to your routine as you become more capable.

Typical workout programs ask you to progress either by adding more weight or more volume via extra reps or sets. Eventually with The Simple Six you will get to the point where a kettlebell is just too light to allow you to properly complete an exercise. When that happens, it's time for a new kettlebell.

However, this shouldn't happen often (think months or even years, not weeks). Buying a new kettlebell should be a celebration. If you're in the market for a new, heavier kettlebell then it means you've put in a ton of practice and hard work. Congratulations!

In the meantime, how do we apply progression to The Simple Six so that it adapts along with you?

Instead of adding more weight or more reps, we're going to add more work by manipulating Time Under Tension (TUT). TUT refers to how long a muscle is under strain during a set of exercise. The longer a rep or set takes to complete, the higher the TUT.

As an exercise starts becoming easier to complete I want you to slow down the movement. Really work to focus on and squeeze the muscles that you're working through the entire range of motion. It's this additional time and focus that works to really up the intensity of an exercise and leads to strength and muscle gains.

So how do we add TUT to an exercise? Let's say that for the push-up you would usually complete a rep with a 1:1:1 tempo. That means you take one second to lower your body, one second to pause at the bottom, and one second to raise your body back to the starting position. If that seems too easy for you then slow it down to a 2:1:2 tempo, then 3:1:3, then 4:1:4, then… you get the idea.

When you can easily complete every set of an (RF) exercise using a 5:1:5 tempo then it's time to increase the weight you're using.

You can make any exercise extremely challenging by increasing TUT so make sure you start out slowly with this technique. Always leave something in the tank for the next day!

Side Note

Slowing down a dynamic movement doesn't make much sense, so TUT doesn't apply to the kettlebell swing. The swing is the one case where I recommend adding reps in order to progress. Once you're completely comfortable performing 5 sets of 10 swings with a given weight start increasing the sets by one rep each week. After you master sets of 20 it's time to level up with a shiny new kettlebell.

17

THE SIMPLE SIX WORKOUT

The Simple Six workout is designed in a five day sequence, meaning it's already custom made to be performed Monday through Friday. However, please don't think this is the only way you can structure your training. If you like training on the weekends, train on the weekends. If you have other commitments or activities on certain days of the week, then move The Simple Six to the next day. If you happen to miss a day here and there don't sweat it, just pick up where you left off the next day. Easy.

The real promise of The Simple Six is that if you follow the program and commit to completing the short workouts as often as you can, then you will see results.

DAY 1

Push-up	1 set of 10 reps
Kettlebell Swing	1 set of 10 reps
Chin-up	1 set
Kettlebell Press	1 set of 10 reps each arm
Goblet Squat (RF)	5 sets of 10 reps
Walking	Option 1, 2, or 3

DAY 2

Goblet Squat	1 set of 10 reps
Kettlebell Swing	1 set of 10 reps
Chin-up	1 set
Kettlebell Press	1 set of 10 reps each arm
Push-up (RF)	5 sets of 10 reps
Walking	Option 1, 2, or 3

DAY 3

Goblet Squat	1 set of 10 reps
Push-up	1 set of 10 reps
Chin-up	1 set
Kettlebell Press	1 set of 10 reps each arm
Kettlebell Swing (RF)	5 sets of 10 reps
Walking	Option 1, 2, or 3

DAY 4

Goblet Squat	1 set of 10 reps
Push-up	1 set of 10 reps
Kettlebell Swing	1 set of 10 reps
Kettlebell Press	1 set of 10 reps each arm
Chin-up (RF)	5 sets
Walking	Option 1, 2, or 3

DAY 5

Goblet Squat	1 set of 10 reps
Push-up	1 set of 10 reps
Kettlebell Swing	1 set of 10 reps
Chin-up	1 set
Kettlebell Press (RF)	5 sets of 10 reps each arm
Walking	Option 1, 2, or 3

So there you have it, The Simple Six workout program. Simple, minimal, elegant.

Thanks for reading, I hope you enjoyed... wait, what's that? You have questions?

"Oh Bother."

-Winnie the Pooh

18

FAQ

YOU DON'T LIST ANY WEIGHTS, ONLY REPS. HOW MUCH WEIGHT SHOULD I BE USING?

The Simple Six program is meant to focus less on weight progression and more on consistency and improved movement. That being said, using the proper weight based on your ability for the kettlebell exercises is still very important.

Because kettlebells are from Russia, and because Russians are crazy (sorry Pavel), kettlebells are measured in poods. A pood is simply a unit of measurement equal to 40 funts. A funt is a Russian pound, so a pood is 40 Russian pounds (about 16 kilograms or 35 pounds). Got it? Good. Moving on.

Russia hasn't used poods as an official unit of measurement for nearly 100 years, so neither will we. Kettlebells are commonly labeled in either kilograms or pounds. While the weights below are rounded slightly, the sizing on kettlebells breaks down like this:

Pounds	Kilograms
9	4
13	6
26	12
35	16
44	20
53	24
62	28
70	32
80	36
88	40
106	48

What size kettlebells are needed for The Simple Six will depend on you as an individual. The stronger you are, the bigger the kettlebell you need.

I recommend that everyone pick two kettlebells that work for them. A lighter kettlebell will be used for the kettlebell press (and 1-arm swings should you ever want to give them a shot), and a heavier bell will be used for the kettlebell swing and the goblet squat.

I also recommend getting kettlebells that you can grow into. Choose a lighter bell that is challenging (but not impossible) for a set of 5 presses and a heavier bell that you have to work to control for a set of 10 swings.

Don't worry if you can't complete the prescribed number of reps with the chosen weights at first, just complete each set with as many reps as you can while maintaining proper form. Before you know it you'll have gained the strength needed for full sets and you won't even remember a time when that kettlebell felt too heavy!

Everyone is different, but the table below should help to give you an idea of what kettlebell might work well as a starting weight for you.

I am a…	Who is…	Light Kettlebell (pounds)	Heavy Kettlebell (pounds)
Woman	A beginner	9, 13	26, 35
Woman	Average Strength	13, 26	35, 44
Woman	Strong	26, 35	44, 53
Man	A beginner	13, 26	35, 44
Man	Average Strength	26, 35	44, 53
Man	Strong	35, 44	53, 70

HOW MANY REPS SHOULD I DO FOR CHIN-UPS?

I'm realistic. I understand that coming into this program not everyone is going to be able to do chin-ups for sets of 10. Many people might struggle to complete a single chin-up. That's great; it means you have a lot of progress to look forward to!

If you can't do a chin-up yet, I want you to start with negative chin-ups. To perform a negative chin-up either jump up or use something like a chair to help you to get into the top position of a chin-up. Pull as hard as you can to try and hold your chin above the bar for a second or two, and then begin lowering yourself slowly down to the bottom position. Let go of the bar, reset, and start over to do additional reps.

Start by doing 1 set of 2 negative chin-ups each day and 5 sets of 1 negative chin-up on the RF day. Increase the number of reps as you get stronger and the negative chin-ups begin to feel easier. Once you are able to do a set of 5 strong, slow negative chin-ups each day, see if you are able to perform your first full chin-up. Getting your first full chin-up is quite an accomplishment and you should be proud of yourself (I'm certainly proud of you!). Now put the negative chin-ups behind you and never look back.

If you can do a chin-up or two, but can't do a full set of 10 then here's the plan. First test yourself by doing a max set of chin-ups. Then subtract one from that number. This is the number of chin-ups you'll use as your starting point. Do 1 set of that number each day, and 5 sets of half that number on RF days.

For example: Let's say you're able to do a max set of 5 chin-ups. Each day you will do 1 set of 4. On RF day you do 5 sets of 2. As you get stronger gradually add reps to both normal and RF days until you are able to do 10 chin-ups for every set.

If you can complete 10 chin-ups for every set on both normal and RF days then congrats, you're a beast. Consider adding weight to the chin-up if you want to keep progressing, otherwise just do your 90 chin-ups a week and consider a side hustle selling tickets to the gun show.

THESE WORKOUTS ARE SO SHORT. IS THERE ENOUGH VOLUME IN THE SIMPLE SIX FOR ME TO BUILD MUSCLE AND GET INTO REALLY GREAT SHAPE?

For decades magazines have been selling bodybuilding style workouts that promise to give you muscle gain, fat loss, six pack abs, and flowing locks of golden hair. Unfortunately, I can't attest to the hair. Some of the workout programs were pretty good, as long as you were able to see through the marketing and apply them to your own goals and abilities.

One of the most popular rep schemes in bodybuilding has always been 3 sets of 10 reps. Let's say you have a bodybuilding style workout you do Monday, Wednesday and Friday. Each workout is made up of five exercises done for 3 sets of 10. That's 150 repetitions per workout, or 450 repetitions per week. Not bad. Bet you'd see results with that right?

Now take a look at The Simple Six. Each day includes a circuit of four exercises done for 1 set of 10 and an RF exercise done for 5 sets of 10. That's 90 repetitions per day. Over the course of 5 days that's, oh my gosh, 450 repetitions. Just like the bodybuilding workout.

The difference is that while each one of the bodybuilding workouts can take 45 minutes to an hour or longer (plus travel time to and from the gym), Simple Six workouts can easily be done from home in a fraction of the time. And because with The Simple Six we're only doing a little each day without going to failure, our workouts will leave you feeling fresh and full of energy, not sore and dreading the walk downstairs after leg day.

WHAT'S THE DEAL WITH WALKING? DO I HAVE TO WALK AT THE END OF MY WORKOUT? HOW FAR OR FOR HOW LONG SHOULD I GO? CAN I LISTEN TO TAYLOR SWIFT ON MY HEADPHONES?

Easy answer - Walk whenever you can, as often as you can, and as far as you can. The amazing thing about walking is that the more you do it, the better you feel. So get out and walk as much as possible every day.

I do know time can be limited though, so I would like to provide a couple of minimums that you should aim to hit.

If you are walking casually, I recommend a minimum of 30 minutes per day. This doesn't have to come at the end of your workout. It doesn't even need to be done consecutively. A couple of very popular methods of getting 30 minutes of walking in a day include splitting it up. 15 minutes in the morning and 15 minutes in the evening, or 10 minutes three times a day when you need a break at work. Your body doesn't notice a difference and it doesn't care, it just wants to move.

Incline walking is harder than casual walking, so you can get the same benefit in less time. The minimum time you should spend incline walking is 15 minutes. I would prefer that you shoot for 30 minutes, or add 15 minutes of casual walking to hit a combined 30 minutes of walking. Still, if time is against you there aren't many 15 minute workouts as effective as walking uphill.

If you've decided to ruck then I'm going to suggest going for mileage instead of time. The reason is that time can be more inconsistent for rucking than for walking without weight. How you feel that day, the amount of weight you're carrying, the terrain you're rucking on... all of these things can affect how fast you're moving during a ruck. So I find it easier to measure rucks in miles. A one-mile ruck is a quick and satisfying weekday workout. If you have the time, 1.5 - 2 miles a day seems to be a real sweet spot for increasing your cardio capacity and amping up the fat loss. I wouldn't go more than 2 miles on a regular day because our goal is to always have something left in the tank for the next day. However, a long hike or a ruck of a few miles or more can be a great way to spend a weekend afternoon!

Remember, these are recommended minimums. 30 minutes of walking is great, an hour of walking is even better. I'd be willing to bet that if you make walking a part of your everyday routine then you'll soon be finding excuses to do it more often.

Finally while I typically prefer to walk without headphones, Tailor Swift is perfectly acceptable. In fact, a recent survey of gym patrons found that 7 in 10 Bro playlists include at least one Tay-Tay track.

I'M USING THE EXERCISES YOU RECOMMEND FOR PEOPLE WHO ARE JUST STARTING OUT, AND IT'S STILL DIFFICULT FOR ME TO GET THROUGH 5 SET OF 10. WHAT SHOULD I DO?

If you are struggling to complete parts of The Simple Six then please scale the workout so that it fits your needs and abilities.

If 5 sets of 10 seems like too much for a given exercise, then lower the number of sets. Complete two or three sets of that exercise and see how you feel over the course of the next week or two. Once you find a comfortable starting point, continue with that workload until it begins to feel too easy. Then, add back another set and re-evaluate.

In time, you will be able to progress to the recommended number of reps and sets and to the recommended exercises.

Don't be discouraged if you find that certain exercises seem to be sticking points. Keep working on them consistently and, in time, everything should come together for you.

Starting slowly and taking your time to cross the finish line is always better than starting out too quickly and never finishing at all.

Side Note

Scaling isn't just for those of us who are new to fitness and working out. If you're feeling down one day or if you're in a real time crunch, then a single circuit consisting of 1 set of each Simple Six exercise is a great way to keep the ball rolling on a day that you otherwise might have skipped. Never forget that consistency outperforms intensity. Those little bits of work can add up to big results over time!

DO YOU HAVE ADDITIONAL QUESTIONS? WANT HELP CUSTOMIZING THE SIMPLE SIX TO YOUR GOALS OR SITUATION?

Reach out and connect with The Simple Six on Facebook @thesimplesix

THANKS SO MUCH, YOU'RE A ROCK STAR!

I'm truly grateful for each and every person who has taken the time to read

The Simple Six

THE EASY WAY TO GET IN SHAPE AND STAY IN SHAPE FOR THE REST OF YOUR LIFE

I hope you found it to be informative and entertaining. Most of all, I hope you give The Simple Six program a chance to change your life the way it has changed mine.

Remember, consistency is the difference between failure and success in almost every aspect of life, but especially so when it comes to your health. So go out and find your passion, stick with it, and live your best life!

NOTE FROM THE AUTHOR

Reviews, rating and shares are gold to authors!

If you've enjoyed this book, please consider showing your appreciation by:

Rating and reviewing The Simple Six on amazon.com

Connecting with The Simple Six on Facebook @thesimplesix

Letting your friends and family know about The Simple Six through social media or good old word of mouth

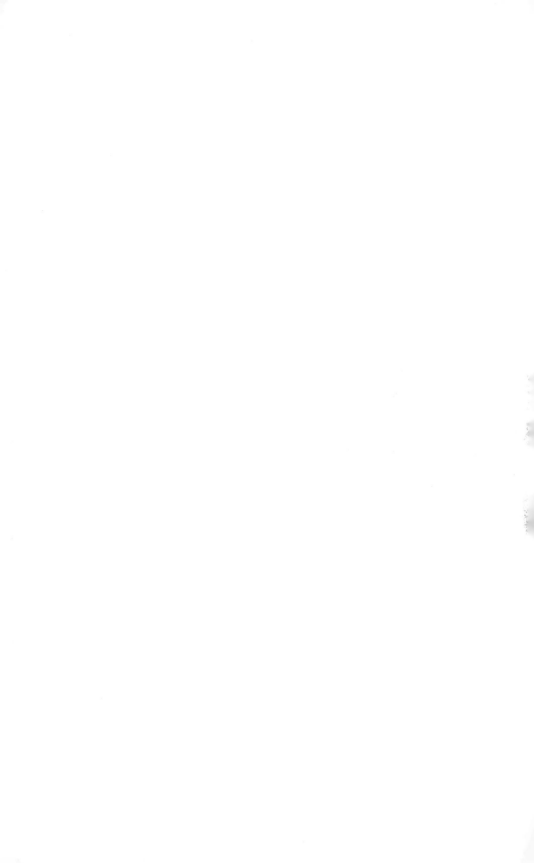

Printed by Amazon Italia Logistica S.r.l.
Torrazza Piemonte (TO), Italy

12498135R00039